The Erectile Dysfunction Solution

Your Complete Guide to Diagnosis, Treatment, and Sexual Performance Enhancement

David H. Levell

Copyright© 2024 David H. Levell All rights reserved.

This work is protected by copyright law and may not be reproduced, distributed, transmitted, displayed, published, or broadcast without the prior written permission of the copyright holder.

Unauthorized use, duplication, or dissemination of this work is strictly prohibited and may result in legal action.

Table Of Content

Introduction

Chapter 1: About Erectile Dysfunction

Chapter 2: Prevention

Chapter 3: How to Improve Your Sexual Performance

Chapter 4: How Is Erectile Dysfunction Diagnosed?

Chapter 5: Treatment Methods

Conclusion

Introduction

II want to thank and congratulate you for downloading the book "How to Last Longer: The Ultimate Guide On How to Last Longer in Bed and Eliminate Erectile Dysfunction Forever".

This book provides tried-and-true procedures and tactics for sleeping longer. Sex is a crucial element of everyone's life, regardless of gender. A healthy sex life balances your life and boosts your confidence and happiness. This helps you and your spouse understand each other better, communicate more effectively, and enjoy life more. We must accept the importance of sexual compatibility. However, having a meaningful personal relationship may be challenging for a variety of reasons, including stress, daily anxieties, health or mental issues, unrealistic expectations, and so on.

This book is a handbook for those who wish to spend more time in bed and get rid of erectile dysfunction. Nowadays, many couples face this issue and find it difficult to discuss. But the good news is that it is fixable if you take it seriously and concentrate on finding a solution. Many guys go through this experience throughout their lives, regardless of age, socioeconomic status, or anything else. Stress impacts us all more than ever, and it is a leading cause of erectile dysfunction.

It is unpleasant and may hurt your ego and self-esteem; nevertheless, keep in mind that it can happen to anybody, and complaining about it will not alter anything. On the contrary, it will exacerbate the situation and negatively impact your relationship. That is why you must take action to understand more about erectile dysfunction and devise a positive solution to the issue. Please don't allow this experience to overwhelm you; instead, strive to be optimistic, get the help you need to get through it and trust in yourself.

Today, an increasing number of men are coping with this problem, which has an impact on their relationships and their whole lives. Yes, we must acknowledge that erectile dysfunction is not an easy topic to discuss since it makes you feel awkward and insignificant. Men are even more hesitant to discuss their concerns, particularly if they are highly personal.

However, nothing can be resolved until action is taken. As uncomfortable and humiliating as it is, men must recognize that erectile dysfunction is a curable illness. It can be improved and addressed if they take it seriously and act responsibly.

And what is the correct thing to do in this situation? Visit a doctor. Seek medical attention from a skilled professional who can assist you in comprehending what you're going through.

Talk to your spouse about your thoughts and concerns, without fear of being seen as weak. On the contrary, this will only strengthen and deepen your friendship. Erectile dysfunction may be both uncomfortable and frustrating for you and your spouse. But there's good news: you can remedy this difficulty. Things will go well if you are dedicated and know what you need to accomplish.

It is also an excellent guide for improving your sexual performance and eliminating erectile dysfunctions.

Thank you again for downloading this book, and I hope you like it!

Chapter 1: About Erectile Dysfunction

EErectile dysfunction is defined as the inability to achieve or maintain a hard adequate erection for sexual intercourse; it is also known as impotence. In most situations, it is only transitory if handled. If you do not take action, your relationship and the quality of your private life may suffer. Fortunately, erectile dysfunction is curable.

If this occurs on occasion, it is not always cause for concern. However, if the issue persists, it may hurt your life, your self-esteem, and your connection with your spouse, as well as cause a great deal of stress. You should also consider the possibility that this is due to an undiagnosed health problem that needs to be treated.

The greatest thing you can do is see a doctor. You must overcome the discomfort of the circumstance and consider your good. The doctor will be able to assist you in identifying the reasons for erectile dysfunction and provide specialist therapy. The sooner you do this, the higher your chances of finding the answer you need. This must be your priority: finding a solution to your problems. Regardless of how humiliating or bothersome it is.

Many men do not see this as an issue until it is too late, and they do not enjoy admitting that they have a problem. But you must understand that erectile dysfunction may be more than just a problem; it might conceal another health issue that you may be unaware of. If you don't take action, it will eventually have an impact on your health and your connection with your spouse. Frustrations may arise, particularly if you are not accustomed to communicating with one another and do not understand one another.

TIf you want to know what's going on, don't ignore the symptoms and see a doctor as soon as possible. Postponing it is not a solution and may exacerbate the situation.

Symptoms of erectile dysfunction

DDifficulty getting an erection

Difficulty maintaining erection

Low libido or desire to have sex

Causes

TThere might be both physical and psychological factors. Many factors may contribute to erectile dysfunction. They may be linked to emotions, hormones, the brain, blood vessels, muscles, or nerves. You should also examine stress and other mental health concerns. Stress is one of the most prevalent psychological factors, influencing both the quality of your sex life and your overall mood. Stress is now a part of our daily lives, and we are unaware of the long-term effects it may have. Because we are unable to separate our business and personal lives, we get irritated, worried, and uptight, which may have an impact on our sexual lives.

Other health concerns may also have an impact on our personal lives, which is why you should take your medicines, follow your doctor's instructions, and strive to live a healthy lifestyle. All of these adjustments may enhance the quality of your life, particularly your one. Ideally, you should examine your health at least once a year, beginning with blood tests, ultrasounds, urine analysis, heart monitoring, and anything else your doctor thinks is necessary.

You should also worry about your nutrition and mental wellness. It is important to take care of yourself, live a tranquil life, and appreciate the time you may spend with your spouse. As you age, your body's demands change and you must be prepared for this. To maintain a healthy lifestyle, you must prioritize yourself, get enough sleep, exercise, and perform your best.

Understandably, your erections will be slower and less hard than they once were, but it doesn't mean you can't enjoy your closeness. There is no need to think such; instead, you should be aware that it may take longer to get and sustain an erection.

However, this does not imply you will be unable to achieve an erection.

As previously said, there are several probable reasons for erectile dysfunction, and the best approach to identify them is to visit your doctor and follow his/her directions. Don't delay; this can't be fixed without expert care, and putting it off isn't in your best interests.

Physical causes

Diabetes

Heart disease

Atherosclerosis

High blood pressure

Metabolic syndrome

Multiple sclerosis

Parkinson's disease

Obesity

Peyronie's disease

Alcohol use

Smoking

Some types of medications

Sleep disorder

Prostate cancer

Injuries or surgeries of the spinal cord or pelvic area Bicycling for a long period

Psychological causes

Stress

Depression

Anxiety

Mental health conditions

Communication problems

Low self-confidence

Complications

Stress

Anxiety

Relationship problems

Low self-esteem

Embarrassment

Unsatisfying sex life

As you can see, erectile dysfunction has several causes and problems. It is also crucial to understand that as you age, you may need more time than normal to get and sustain an erection. This disease does become worse as you get older. It most often affects males over the age of 50, however, this is not always the case. Also, just because you take longer to obtain an erection does not indicate you have erectile dysfunction.

The greatest thing you can do is consult a doctor, who will accurately diagnose you and suggest remedies to your condition. Unfortunately, many men hesitate to do so because they are ashamed, and instead prefer to diagnose and cure themselves using the Internet. This is highly risky and may endanger your health. Online diagnosis cannot substitute a physical examination and any other tests that your doctor may want. As a result, it is preferable to disregard the humiliation and seek medical attention right once.

Your health should be your priority. Nothing can be more vital than that, and you must recognize that the doctor is the only one who can assist you. If you opt to take medicine without seeing a doctor, you put yourself in danger, which is not in your best interests. Instead of taking unnecessary chances with your health, it's best to seek professional assistance.

We understand how painful it may be to acknowledge that you are experiencing erection problems, but try to talk with your spouse and work together to find a solution. You are not alone in this; your spouse plays a crucial role, and you can depend on her support. Talking with your spouse is vital because it allows you to view things from a new perspective.

Most likely, erectile dysfunction is a transient condition in your life, but if you don't address it, it may affect you in a variety of ways. Many guys suffering from erectile dysfunction feel they can manage the problem on their own, that they are OK, and do not want any assistance. Yes, it is difficult to acknowledge how this might affect your sexual life, self-confidence, connection with your spouse, self-esteem, and so on. But you are the only one who can overcome it and make things work.

The first thing you should do is consult a doctor to determine if you have erectile dysfunction. Perhaps you will see that this is not the case and that the issue lies elsewhere. Don't allow this issue consume your whole life; instead, take action and concentrate on determining the reason and solution to your problem. The sooner you do it, the better the outcome. Do not hesitate or waste time, since this will not affect the diagnosis.

Chapter 2: Prevention

Preventing erectile dysfunction is both simple and challenging. You must not just satisfy your sexual urge but also care for yourself from a variety of perspectives. Your libido or urge for sex is not something that happens on its own; it can be controlled and influenced, at least somewhat. As a result, when you are unhappy, angered, disturbed, or depressed, you are unlikely to experience the desire for sex, resulting in a delayed erection. On the contrary, if you had a wonderful day, if you are cheerful, joyous, and hopeful, you are more likely to be in the mood for sex and to get a hard and powerful erection in a short time.

This implies that your mind and body are inextricably linked, and they must be in harmony. That is why psychological factors are just as significant as physical ones in the case of erectile dysfunction. If you are under stress, your body may express this via an erection issue.

However, a physical cause might be the primary explanation. You might have an undiagnosed ailment, or certain drugs could interfere with your libido and cause erection problems. As you can see, many factors may have an impact on your sexual life, but you must prioritize yourself and choose the best answer for your situation.

Can erectile dysfunction be prevented? To a large part, the answer is yes; it is preventable. If you take good care of yourself, attempt to live a healthy lifestyle, exercise, and avoid stress, you have a good chance of having a normal, enjoyable sexual relationship with your spouse. We already know that erectile dysfunction may be an indication of another condition, therefore the healthier you are, the more likely you are to never face this problem.

You must maintain your health for as long as possible, whether you are twenty or seventy. Do not be disappointed, and do not let despair overpower you. Do your best to live a healthy lifestyle and be happy, and you will find that it will benefit you much. A healthy body cultivates a healthy mind, which leads to a healthier existence. The many parts of our lives are interconnected, and we must strike a balance in all of them.

You may avoid erectile dysfunction by taking care of yourself and being physically active. Physical activity is essential for your sex life. The more active you are, the greater your sexual experience will be. Other crucial factors include a balanced diet, enough sleep, a happy mindset, and stress reduction. All of these factors lead to a fulfilling sexual life.

Self-care is crucial at any age, not just when you're young. If you want to appreciate life to the fullest, you must do so, particularly as you become older. But how precisely can you avoid erectile dysfunction? Here are some practical recommendations you should follow:

Live a healthy lifestyle.

Although this may seem insignificant, it has a huge impact on your sexual health. You must prioritize your physical and mental well-being. Consider making good adjustments, such as:

Losing Weight.

This is the leading cause of erectile dysfunction. Not to mention that smoking endangers your life, drains your energy, and might affect your libido. Obesity is a sickness that must be addressed. So, try to concentrate on a healthy strategy to lose weight. Consult a nutritionist to create a balanced and individualized diet based on your health issues and other drugs.

Exercise regularly.

This is an excellent strategy for weight loss, but you should continue to exercise even after you have lost the weight. You may go on a run, attend the gym, swim, work out at home, or do anything else. Exercising benefits your physical health keeps you youthful, and generates endorphins, which make you joyful and give you energy.

Stop smoking.

This affects both your lungs and your general health. Simultaneously, it has the potential to produce erectile dysfunction. Quitting smoking will make you feel a lot healthier.

Don't overreact to alcohol use.

A glass or two of wine provides numerous advantages for your brain's health and happiness, but if you overdo it, the benefits turn into hazards.

Sleep soundly.

Do not underestimate the value of sleep in your life. If you want to remain healthy and have enough energy for the next day, you need to get 7-8 hours of excellent quality sleep every night. Sleep issues are a common cause of erectile dysfunction, so don't overlook this component. If you are having difficulty sleeping at night, you should contact a doctor since this is a simple problem to fix.

Manage your illnesses.

If you have a chronic ailment, you must keep it under control by taking your medications and doing your best to care for yourself. This enables you to sustain functioning erections for a longer period. You may potentially be suffering from an undiagnosed ailment, thus it is recommended that you get yearly testing to assess your health.

Blood sugar.

Reduce your sugar intake, since it might affect your erections and raise your risk of obesity and heart disease. Eat a nutritious diet rich in fruits and vegetables, and drink lots of water.

High blood pressure is another risk factor, so aim to keep it at a reasonable range. Reduce your salt intake and remember to hydrate yourself.

Maintain cholesterol under control.

High cholesterol is harmful to your health and may result from an unhealthy diet and lifestyle. You may lessen it by taking medication and changing your diet.

Prostate Disorders.

This may be another reason for erectile dysfunction. You should examine your prostate once a year to ensure that everything is OK. This lowers the risk of prostate cancer and enhances erections.

Mental health is another risk factor for erectile dysfunction. Many individuals feel that erectile dysfunction is caused by a medical ailment, thus they do not consider mental health. However, studies have proven that mental equilibrium is essential for your sexual life and the quality of your erections. It's no surprise that stress reduces your desire for sex and may even induce temporary erectile dysfunction. To maintain good mental health, attempt the following:

Reduce stress as much as possible. Try relaxing methods such as meditation and breathing control.

Do not let anxiousness overcome you.

Many guys with erectile dysfunction feel frightened and embarrassed of themselves. But what you must do is be strong, take charge of the situation, and combat anxiousness. Try to remain cheerful, have a good attitude, find a solution, and avoid letting negative ideas impact you.

Depression reduces the quality of your sex life and erections. At the same time, it lowers your self-esteem and causes you to concentrate on the bad aspects of your life. As a result, do not be afraid to see a doctor and seek treatment for depression.

Communication.

Effective communication between you and your spouse may greatly improve matters. This enables you to communicate with each other and be honest. At the very least, knowing that your spouse supports and understands you is beneficial psychologically. If you want a wonderful relationship, learn how to communicate with each other, share your thoughts, and listen to what your spouse has to say.

Pay attentive attention to what your companion is saying.

Express your emotions without harming the other person.

Focus on finding a solution together.

Talk to each other about your issues.

Check your testosterone levels.

It is commonly known that testosterone levels drop at the age of 50, which might influence your sexual life. A low testosterone level may be the cause of poor libido, low stamina, a lack of energy to accomplish basic tasks, and problems with erections. Consult your doctor for treatment options.

Many guys assume that they don't need to do anything to have a successful romantic relationship. This could work if you're twenty, but as you get older, things begin to change. As a result, you must recognize the importance of your health and take your own well-being seriously. A wonderful sexual performance is stunning, but it does not occur if you are overweight or sedentary. You must be active in your relationship, striving to improve yourself every day and connecting with your spouse.

Preventing erectile dysfunction is a lifelong process that cannot be completed in a matter of days. You must grasp this and strive every day to enhance the quality of your life, not only your sexual life. This is only one of the many advantages of leading a healthy lifestyle. Perform several tests regularly to assess your general health and determine what you can do to improve the areas you dislike.

Also, don't overlook your mental health; it's critical to strike a balance between your body and your head. Try to lessen stress, connect with your spouse, concentrate on the good things in your life, and have a cheerful attitude.

Chapter 3: How to Improve Your Sexual Performance

Many guys are concerned about their sexual performance. They want to endure longer, keep their partners happy, and be recognized for their talents. There is nothing wrong with it. Everyone wants to feel good, to enjoy themselves, to be free and joyful. But what are your expectations for your sexual performance? Do you want to gratify your partner? Do you want to do better than the prior time? What is your goal? Sexual performance is about more than just oneself, therefore "measuring" it might be more difficult since various elements must be considered.

Who determines your sexual performance? Is it you, or your partner? Or both? You should answer these questions to determine what you need to accomplish. Men usually describe sexual performance as the time of intercourse. The longer they survive, the better they believe everything is. And this is somewhat correct. But time is not everything. You may enhance your performance in a variety of ways, based on your partner's demands and your expectations.

First and foremost, try to relax.

Many guys are enamored with the concept of living longer. And, certainly, women must acknowledge that although this is essential, it is not everything. Other important factors are your partner's attention, physical contact, the connection between you two, your wants, and your expectations. Good communication is the key to resolving your sexual issues. You cannot increase your sexual performance if you are unable to communicate with each other and do not understand what your spouse wants.

Try to concentrate on pleasing your partner

This entails chatting to her and learning about her desires, needs, likes, and dislikes. This should be the initial step. Then you may concentrate on staying longer. There is some practical general advice you can follow to increase your sexual performance, such as watching your nutrition, exercising, and lowering stress. You will see the change within a short period.

The good thing is that you can always enhance your sexual performance if you want to. There is no age restriction; you only need to know yourself and your partner. Yes, having erectile dysfunction is bothersome and frustrating, but it does not imply your romantic life is over. Consider it merely a stepping stone to conquer.

If you understand what you need to accomplish, your sexual performance will improve, which will pleasure both you and your partner. Here are some suggestions to increase your sexual performance:

Try to relax. Stop doubting yourself and fretting about your erections. This adds tension to your shoulders, which will impact your erections. So, try to relax and enjoy the time you get to spend with your lover. Don't think about anything else; just live in the present moment and forget about anything else. Try to teach your mind to dwell in the present moment, rather than wandering about aimlessly.

Concentrate on cardiovascular exercise.

This enhances both your health and sexual performance. You do not need to spend all day at the gym; thirty minutes every day is plenty. Swimming and jogging are excellent ways to increase your libido and enhance erections. You may also participate in different sports based on your interests. The most essential thing is to exercise, to develop both your body and your mind simultaneously. This helps you feel good and healthy.

Include the following foods in your diet: garlic, onions, bananas, chilies and peppers, omega-3 fatty acids, eggs, and vitamin B1. These are beneficial to your health and may considerably enhance your sexual experience.

Get some sunlight. This improves your mood and increases your sexual drive. So don't remain home; instead, go out and enjoy yourself. Fresh air is excellent for enhancing libido, particularly on warm days and nights. Consider taking a trip with your lover to a hot place where you can put everything you've learned in this book into practice.

Masturbation might make you stay longer in bed. Before having sex with your lover, you may practice masturbating.

Connect with your partner.

A fantastic sexual experience includes both of you. As a result, don't concentrate only on your performance, since this will make your partner feel irrelevant. Focus on relaxing her and doing things she enjoys. Things will improve if you don't continually obsess about how to live longer.

Visit a sexologist.

This may be an excellent method to learn more about yourself, your sexuality, and how you might enhance your relationships. You may bring your partner with you to discuss your issues and expectations. There is nothing to be embarrassed of. Consider that these folks have to do this every day and have most likely heard a variety of things over their employment. So, try to be honest and consider this as a chance to learn new things and address your difficulties.

Experience new things.

Routine is the enemy of a fulfilling sexual life, so try your best to prevent it. Try changing your location, your clothing, role-playing, or anything else that will discourage you from falling into a habit. Discuss your areas for improvement with your spouse and try your best to reach an agreement. A connection requires time and communication; it is not easy to accomplish or comprehend.

Boost your self-confidence.

Women are more prone to have low self-confidence than males, however, this may happen to either gender. If you don't believe in yourself, if you're worried about how to live longer and can't relax, you'll simply make matters worse. To boost your self-esteem, strive to maintain a good attitude; do something for yourself, such as purchase a great jacket or new perfume, or trim your hair differently. See what makes you feel good about yourself since this will boost your self-esteem and sexual performance.

Try various positions.

To break out of the ordinary and explore new methods to enjoy your private life, try out various positions. Talk to your girlfriend about her dreams and what she wants to explore. Tell her about your desires and try new things. Establish a line that you are not permitted to cross, according to your preferences.

Try Kegel exercises.

They have several advantages and may be performed by both men and women. You may perform them anywhere: at home, while driving, while cooking, at work, or anyplace else. Tighten your pelvic muscles and hold the tension for a few seconds before releasing. You should repeat at least ten times for each set, and you may perform many sets each day. This gradually enhances your erections and allows you to maintain control for extended periods.

Be patient.

If you are having a tough time at work, allow yourself time to resolve the issue. Do not anticipate rapid solutions and avoid becoming gloomy. Instead, concentrate on finding a solution to your issue rather than criticizing yourself. Even if you decide to visit a doctor, don't expect anything to change within a week. It takes time to figure out what's wrong and what you should do, and you need to know you can rely on your partner's support.

Never give up!

It might be irritating to spend time trying to figure out what's causing erectile dysfunction. You may need to attempt many therapies but don't give up. It is only an issue of time and determination to achieve. If you are not fortunate enough to get the correct therapy the first time around, trial and error may be unavoidable.

You may improve your libido by taking supplements or eating certain foods, but only if your doctor recommends it. Don't use supplements without contacting a doctor since they might produce a variety of negative effects and interact with other drugs you're taking. They may have an impact on your heart and body's overall function. As much as you'd want to think they're the solution to your issues, this is seldom true. Don't fool around with your health. If you wish to prevent this, always consult your doctor before taking supplements.

Chapter 4: How Is Erectile Dysfunction Diagnosed?

Erectile dysfunction is a particularly uncomfortable topic for guys. It is difficult to accept that you are having difficulties in your personal life and that you need assistance. But there's nothing to be embarrassed of since this isn't your fault. Or independent of you. Something causes this circumstance, and it takes time to figure out what it is. Sometimes it's a sickness, stress, or anything else. However, without a diagnosis, you don't know what to do. Stop putting it off, attempt to figure out what's causing it, and come up with a viable solution. The sooner the better.

When you are experiencing erection troubles, you must consult a doctor. Only an expert can assist you in resolving the issue. However, this may be a sensitive subject for males who are terrified and humiliated by the physical examination. We understand how terrible it may be, but it is the only way to get a diagnosis and receive appropriate therapy. Remember that you aim to concentrate on a solution. Remember that the doctor is there to assist you with your medical experience; he or she will know how to make you feel better and more comfortable.

It is preferable if you know what to anticipate during the medical consultation, therefore we will provide you with some important information.

On a piece of paper, write down all of the symptoms you encountered, even some that do not seem to be connected to this problem: low libido, difficulty getting and keeping an erection, poor self-esteem, exhaustion, anxiety, sleep disturbance, etc.

Write down the main events in your life that have occurred lately, such as a job change, the loss of a close relative, or troubles with your relationship.

List all of the drugs you're taking for your ailments, including vitamins and supplements.

Prepare a list of questions to ask the doctor.

You are welcome to bring your spouse if you feel comfortable doing so.

It is preferable to have a list of questions to ask the doctor, which you may prepare before the consultation. Prepare yourself before going to the doctor; consider what you want to know about the reasons, investigation techniques, and potential treatments. Get educated before visiting the doctor so that you may get the most out of your consultation. Here are a few potential questions:

What might be the source of this issue?

What tests should I run?

How long does it take to resolve erectile dysfunction?

What are the therapy options?

Are there any physical restrictions?

You can also expect your doctor to ask you questions about your medical history, past ailments, stressful situations, relationship with your spouse, sexual life, and current concerns. Some questions may seem to be extremely personal, but keep in mind that they are merely intended to determine the source of erectile dysfunction; try not to take things personally or get angry about it. You should be open and honest while answering these questions since they are only intended to assist you.

The physical examination.

The doctor will examine your penis, testicles, and nerves. It won't be painful, just uncomfortable. Fortunately, this will only take a few minutes, so try to remain as comfortable as possible and believe that it will soon be done. It is not as difficult as some men imagine, nor is it unpleasant.

Additional testing.

Typically, the doctor may order blood tests to determine your testosterone levels, as well as any potential heart disease, diabetes, or other conditions. If your doctor expressly requests them, you may complete them before your consultation.

Urine test.

To rule out any health issues or infections, you will most likely need to do a urine test.

Ultrasound.

This procedure is conducted on the penis' blood arteries. It is recommended that you get this ultrasound to see if you have any blood flow issues. This test may be performed with an injection to induce an erection and improve blood flow.

Erection Test

This test entails wearing a specific gadget around your penis at night before going to bed. This is used to determine the frequency and intensity of your nocturnal erections.

Electrocardiogram.

This allows the doctor to determine whether anything is amiss with your heart.

Psychological examination.

In addition to the physical test, you will most likely be required to undergo a psychological examination. This entails completing certain questions to determine if you have anxiety or depression. This may be done by your doctor or another professional physician.

Following the medical consultation, your doctor will be able to determine if your erectile dysfunction is caused by a physical or psychological component. At the same time, he or she will recommend the best treatment option for your instance.

Chapter 5: Treatment Methods

The good news is that erectile dysfunction is treatable. If you are willing to see a doctor and follow his/her instructions, you will be able to solve this frustrating problem. There are many treatment methods available nowadays for erectile dysfunction and you should choose the one that best suits you together with your doctor. You need to take into account your previous health conditions, your overall health, your medications, and your preferences, as well.

The doctor is there to help you choose the best treatment option; however, if you don't succeed the first time, don't give up, try a different treatment until you succeed. Regarding the oral treatment method, it is important to know that you have to take these pills for a limited period, not your entire life. If they don't seem to work after a while, maybe you should have another talk with your doctor and choose a different treatment. As we have already said, you can't know from the beginning what it is going to work in your case, you just have to try until you find something suitable for you.

Erectile dysfunction responds to numerous treatment methods, according to the primary cause. It is advisable to follow the doctor's guidelines and ask for a second opinion if you want to be sure of your options. If you are suffering from other health conditions, your doctor will take that into account and prescribe a personalized treatment. He/she must explain to you about the risks and benefits of each treatment type and also consider your preferences. You can opt for a treatment method together with your doctor and, maybe, your partner.

Oral medications

This is the first option for erectile dysfunction and it works in the case of many men, as long as they don't interfere with other medications or health conditions.

Among these medications, are:

Avanafil

Vardenafil

Tadalafil

Sildenafil

Their action is to relax the muscles in the penis, which increases the blood flow and helps you have an erection. Your doctor will establish how long you should take these oral pills. Remember you have to come for a second consult after one to two months; if nothing changes until then, it's time to think of a different treatment method.

Possible side effects of oral medications are:

Headaches

Visual changes

Stomach upset

Nasal congestion

Flushing

It is also important to know that it may take a while for a certain medication to be effective, so you need to be patient. More than that, you may need to try several types of medications before finding something that works for you. It takes time and you need to be aware of it. But don't give up.

Self-injections with alprostadil.

This is another treatment method, which involves injecting a substance at the base of your penis. The immediate result of this injection is a strong erection, which will last about an hour.

Possible side effects:

Bleeding

Prolonged erection

Fibrous tissue at the injection place

Urethral suppository with alprostadil.

This involves placing a suppository with alprostadil inside your penis, more specifically in the penile urethra. This is done using a special instrument. The result is a strong erection, which appears in the following ten minutes and lasts for about thirty-sixty minutes.

Possible side effects:

Bleeding

Pain

Fibrous tissue inside your penis

Testosterone replacement therapy

This is another popular method used for treating erectile dysfunction. It is not painful, it can increase your libido and improve your sexual life. But the results do not appear immediately and the side effects are not very pleasant, so you will have to wait a while before noticing the changes and overcoming some of the side effects.

Possible side effects:

Penis aching

Breast enlargement

Acne

Urination problems

Scarring

Penis pumps

More and more men prefer to use a penis pump to have an erection. This is a tube placed over your penis, which sucks the air inside of it. When you have an erection, you have to place a tension ring around your penis, to hold the blood flow and keep it firm. The erection typically lasts for about fifteen-thirty minutes and you have to remove the ring after intercourse. This is not a very pleasant method, but it works for the majority of cases, so it can work for you, too.

Possible side effects:

Restriction of ejaculation

Penis bruise

Cold penis

Penile implants

This is another method to treat erectile dysfunction. This involves placing devices into both sides of your penis, under surgery. Doctors usually use inflatable or semi-rigid rods. Inflatable rods help you control when you will have an erection and for how long; semi rigid rods can help you keep your penis firm, but still bendable. However, you should know that this method is recommended only after you have unsuccessfully tried all the other methods. It has some risks; therefore, you have to be sure you want to do this.

Possible side effects:

Infection

Other surgery complications

Surgery of the blood vessel

This is also a treatment method that requires surgery; therefore, there are some risks you need to take into account. The surgery is realized with the help of a vascular stenting or with a bypass procedure. This surgery can be performed when the blood vessels are leaking or are obstructed and this leads to erectile dysfunction. It is a quite rare case, but it can happen.

Possible side effects:

Surgery complications

Pain

Besides these treatment methods, there are also natural remedies, which can improve your erections and increase your desire for sex.

Panax, Ginseng, and Rhodiola Roseola are used for naturally treating erectile dysfunction.

DHEA (Dehydroepiandrosterone) is a natural hormone that can be converted to estrogen and testosterone. You can take it as a dietary supplement

L-arginine is also very effective for erectile dysfunction. Some studies suggest that L-Arginine with Pycnogenol can significantly improve sexual life after two to three months.

Acupuncture is a controversial treatment, which had great results for some men and poor results for others. It might work for you if you are willing to try it.

Zinc supplements can improve your erectile dysfunction, especially if your body is low on zinc.

Remember that you need to try more possibilities before finding the best solution for you, in case you don't succeed from the very first time. That is why you need to talk to your doctor and discuss the treatment. Try to be optimistic and focus on what you have to do, rather than spend your time getting frustrated or upset. Fortunately, erectile dysfunction can be treated, you just need to find the best solution. Don't take any supplements or try any new treatments without the approval of your doctor.

Conclusion

Erectile dysfunction can be a very difficult time in your life if you allow it to control your life and change who you are. But you shouldn't allow this to happen; on the contrary, you have to fight to overcome this moment, to maintain a positive attitude, and to find a balance. Even if your self-confidence has been affected by this situation, this doesn't mean your entire life will be like this.

You need to find support, to talk to your partner and your doctor; you can also see a therapist to help you cope with this difficult experience. As hard as it may seem, you need to move forward and focus on yourself and your partner. As you have already seen, erectile dysfunction is treatable; therefore, you just need to find adequate treatment.

At the same time, try to change your lifestyle, lead a healthy life, be positive, and enjoy your life, together with your partner. Focus on improving the relationship between the two of you, on creating a balance between your body and your mind, and on being happy. Erectile dysfunction is a temporary condition and you will be able to overcome it if you are patient and persevering.

Do the best you can to improve the quality of your life and changes will be visible in a short period. Try to connect with your partner, with yourself, and remember that you have to be strong, to succeed. Keep a positive attitude and you will make it!

www.ingramcontent.com/pod-product-compliance
Lightning Source LLC
Chambersburg PA
CBHW071955210526
45479CB00003B/950